How To Treat And Cure Arthritis

339 Great Tips To Get Relief From Arthritis Pain

ADAM COLTON

Published by BizMove
www.bizmove.com

ISBN: 1978368933
ISBN- 978-1978368934

Table of Contents

1 Arthritis Fact Sheet   5

2 339 Great Tips To Get Relief From Arthritis   11
   Pain

1. Arthritis Fact Sheet

What is it?

"Arthritis" literally means joint inflammation. Although joint inflammation is a symptom or sign rather than a specific diagnosis, the term arthritis is often used to refer to any disorder that affects the joints. Joints are places where two bones meet, such as your elbow or knee.

There are different types of arthritis. In some diseases in which arthritis occurs, other organs, such as your eyes, heart, or skin, can also be affected.

Fortunately, current treatments allow most people with arthritis to lead active and productive lives.

Points To Remember About Arthritis

- "Arthritis" means joint inflammation. Although joint inflammation is a symptom or sign rather than a specific diagnosis, the term arthritis is often used to refer to any disorder that affects the joints.

- There are many types of arthritis, including ankylosing spondylitis, gout, juvenile arthritis, osteoarthritis, psoriatic arthritis, reactive arthritis, and rheumatoid arthritis.
- Medications and surgery can treat arthritis.
- Activities that can help reduce symptoms at home include exercise; hot and cold therapies; relaxation therapies; splints and braces; and assistive devices.

"Arthritis" literally means joint inflammation. Although joint inflammation is a symptom or sign rather than a specific diagnosis, the term arthritis is often used to refer to any disorder that affects the joints. Joints are places where two bones meet, such as your elbow or knee.

There are different types of arthritis. In some diseases in which arthritis occurs, other organs, such as your eyes, heart, or skin, can also be affected.

Fortunately, current treatments allow most people with arthritis to lead active and productive lives.

What are the types?

There are several types of arthritis. Common ones include:

- **Ankylosing Spondylitis** is arthritis that affects the spine. It often involves redness, heat, swelling, and pain in the spine or in the joint where the bottom of the spine joins the pelvic bone.
- **Gout** is caused by crystals that build up in the joints. It usually affects the big toe, but many other joints may be affected.
- **Juvenile Arthritis** is the term used to describe arthritis in children. Arthritis is caused by inflammation of the joints.
- **Osteoarthritis** usually comes with age and most often affects the fingers, knees, and hips. Sometimes osteoarthritis follows a joint injury. For example, you might have badly injured your knee when young and develop arthritis in your knee joint years later.
- **Psoriatic Arthritis** can occur in people who have psoriasis (scaly red and white skin patches). It affects the skin, joints, and areas where tissues attach to bone.
- **Reactive Arthritis** is pain or swelling in a joint that is caused by an infection in your body. You may also have red, swollen eyes and a swollen urinary tract.
- **Rheumatoid arthritis** happens when the body's own defense system doesn't work properly. It affects joints and bones (often of the hands and feet), and may also affect internal organs and

systems. You may feel sick or tired, and you may have a fever.

What are the symptoms?

Symptoms of arthritis can include:

- Pain, redness, heat, and swelling in your joints.
- Trouble moving around.
- Fever.
- Weight loss.
- Breathing problems.
- Rash or itch.

These symptoms may also be signs of other illnesses.

What causes it?

There are probably many genes that make people more likely to have arthritis. Research has found some of these genes.

If you have the gene linked with arthritis, something in your environment—such as a virus or injury—may trigger the condition.

Is there a test?

To diagnosis you with arthritis or another rheumatic disease, your doctor may:

- Ask you about your medical history.
- Give you a physical exam.
- Take samples for a laboratory test.
- Take x-rays.

How is it treated?

There are many treatments that can help relieve pain and help you live with arthritis. You should talk to your doctor about the best treatments for you, which can include:

- **Medications** to relieve pain, slow the condition, and prevent further damage.
- **Surgery** to repair joint damage or relieve pain.

Who treats it?

Doctors who diagnose and treat arthritis and other rheumatic disease include:

- A general practitioner, such as your family doctor.
- A rheumatologist, who treats arthritis and other diseases of the bones, joints, and muscles.

Living With It

There are many things you can do to help you live with arthritis and other rheumatic diseases, including:

- Take your medications when and how you're supposed to.
- Exercise to reduce joint pain and stiffness. It also helps with losing weight, which reduces stress on the joints. You should speak to your doctor about a safe, well-rounded exercise program.
- Use heat and cold therapies to reduce joint pain and swelling.
- Try relaxation therapy to help reduce pain by learning ways to relax your muscles.
- Use splints and braces to support weakened joints or allow them to rest. You should see your doctor to make sure your splint or brace fits well.
- Use assistive devices, such as a cane or shoe insert, to ease pain when walking. Other devices can help you open a jar, close zippers, or hold pencils.

2. 339 Great Tips To Get Relief From Arthritis Pain

Is arthritis taking over your life? There are a lot of people that have a hard time due to the decreased capabilities and pain caused by arthritis, and a lot of them are not aware of the remedies and treatments that are out there. Even without medication, you could be doing something about your arthritis with effective measures. These below suggestions will help you deal with arthritis in your life.

1. Be sure to get enough exercise and that you are doing the right kinds of exercise. People with arthritis should choose exercises that support and strengthen the joints, such as swimming, instead of exercises that damage them, such as running. Failing to exercise can also increase joint stiffness and pain.

2. Arthritis is becoming more and more common! If you notice that you have pain, swelling, or stiffness around your joints, it is important that you see your doctor right away! This could be a sign of arthritis, and if that is the case, you want

treatment to begin as soon as possible. Make sure, you also, ask your doctor what kind of arthritis it is. This will be helpful when getting the proper treatment!

3. Eat the right supplements. Omega 3 fish oils have been shown to greatly reduce inflammation and swelling of joints, as well as help to increase flexibility. Make sure you are taking these supplements as they are prescribed, and you will quickly find yourself able to do the tasks you were worried you would not be able to do.

4. Cool down your joints and stop physical activity if you start feeling arthritis pain. Rest in a cool environment and use cold packs or mists of cold water to help reduce the pain and swelling caused by injury. Make sure to rest the injured joints and let them have time to get back to fighting order before using them for any difficult tasks.

5. See a doctor to find out exactly what type of arthritis you have if you feel you are suffering from arthritic symptoms. There are over one hundred different types of arthritis and knowing your specific type can help you learn how to help take care of yourself more effectively.

6. Walking is an activity that helps arthritis in many aspects. Not only does it help your body to release any tensions it may have, but it also helps by stretching out weak joints and muscles. If it is possible, try to talk a 20 to 30 minute walk every day.

7. Electrical stimulation can be a great treatment for osteoarthritis, but consult your doctor about the pros and cons. This treatment will make the swelling reduce right away and make the pain disappear.

8. Buy helpful equipment. Having the correct tools can make your job a whole lot easier. Available products include specialized knives, can openers, attachments for zippers and shoe horns, each designed so an arthritis sufferer can do daily tasks without additional help. Consider surrounding yourself with these useful tools as a means to make your life a bit easier.

9. It is essential that you talk to a physician when your symptoms start appearing and that you begin treatment right away if you need it. You can reduce the damage to your joints from arthritis by getting your start against the effects early. Get started by talking to a doctor and finding out what treatment is best for you.

10. Be sure to drink enough water. Always choose water over other drinks, and drink as often as you can. Avoid beverages that will cause dehydration, such as anything that contains caffeine.

11. Do as much reading and researching as you can to learn about all the new innovations in arthritis therapy, both in the mainstream world of medicine and in a vast variety of alternative therapies. By knowing what's available to you, you will be able to create the most effective and creative therapy plan to address your arthritis pain needs.

12. Be sure to visit your doctor if you experience a strain, sprain or significant bruising. Your doctor can examine the injury to be sure it is not too serious and recommend the best treatment for proper recovery. Protect yourself by allowing a doctor to treat your injuries, even if they do not immediately seem severe.

13. Juvenile rheumatoid arthritis may go into remission for years and may seem to be cured; however, it can come back in full force at any time. For this reason, it is very important for young people with juvenile rheumatoid arthritis

to continue exercising and following a proper, anti-inflammatory, weight control diet. This will help control pain and symptoms if/when the disease returns.

14. Beating the fatigue associated with rheumatoid arthritis isn't easy, but there are ways to keep it under control. For example, stick to a schedule every day - even on the weekend - as to when you go to bed and when you get up in the morning. This will help insure you get a good night's sleep every day.

15. Snacking is a great way to get the nutrients your body needs to keep active, even if arthritis is trying to hold you back. Eat healthy snacks like seeds, fruit, nuts or protein bars. These types of foods will give you an energy boost, without adding a lot of sodium or sugar in your body.

16. Make sure you get enough sleep. Not sleeping enough will cause fatigue and stress, which can make arthritis worst. You should get at least eight hours of sleep every night and keep a regular schedule. Do not hesitate to take naps during the day if you feel you need to.

17. Avoid putting too much pressure on your joints. Even if they are not hurting, you should still

avoid lifting heavy things or typing on a keyboard for too long. You will have to make conscious efforts at first to protect your joints but very soon everything will become a habit.

18. Ice packs or heat pads are great to relieve joint pain. For the best results, alternate between the hot and cold applications. Consult with a doctor, as he or she might have additional tips for using temperature to soothe arthritis pain.

19. Surprisingly, controlled alcohol consumption won't worsen the effects of your arthritis. Surprisingly, these studies instead came to the conclusion that drinking moderately could reduce the intensity of symptoms.

20. If your arthritis pain is affecting your sleep, try getting a warm bath with bath salts in the evening. The bath and salts will soothe your muscles and ease arthritis pain; you'll be able to find sleep more easily and sleep that much longer.

21. See a doctor to find out exactly what type of arthritis you have if you feel you are suffering from arthritic symptoms. There are over one hundred different types of arthritis and knowing

your specific type can help you learn how to help take care of yourself more effectively.

22. Find a support group. Suffering from arthritis can make you feel like an invisible and lonely victim, even when you are not. Joining a support group of others who have the same condition can help you feel better about it, as well as give you a way to share ideas for coping.

23. Add ginger to your food. Ginger is well known for relieving inflammation and stiffness, so adding a few grams a day to your foods can help you reap the benefits of this healthy plant. Ginger and honey drinks are the best method, as honey also gives some of the same benefits.

24. If you have been having trouble turning door knobs, consider having your door hardware switched out for handles instead of knobs. When you are dealing with arthritis flare ups, you can use your elbow and forearm to do the work of opening the door saving your hands the trouble.

25. Never wear high heels. Women who suffer from arthritis should stay far away from these shoes, as they put extra stress on the ankles and knees. Wearing these can actually cause tears in the tendons surrounding joints, which will only

worsen any inflammation and pain that already exists in the area.

26. Black Cohosh can help relieve the pain and other symptoms of arthritis. It works on eliminating the inflammation associated with arthritis and can be helpful in reducing other neurological pain, as well as being beneficial for the nervous system. Try Black Cohosh if you desire to live pain-free and engage in activities during the day.

27. One if the big factors that has been linked to arthritis and decreasing your overall health is smoking. Do not smoke. This lifestyle factor has been associated and known to cause severe joint damage when coupled with people who have arthritis. So improve your health and make your joints feel better by not smoking.

28. Sometimes, the treatments that your doctor offers for arthritis can be assisted and enhanced with alternative treatments such as hydrotherapy, yoga, hot and cold therapy or some herbal or dietary supplements. Be sure to ask your doctor about alternative treatments that will help you make the most of your arthritis care.

29. You will never know if alternative treatments for arthritis work for you until you try them. There is a whole world of therapy, exercise and alternative herbal and supplemental treatment to explore. Most forms of alternative therapy are good for your general health as well as your arthritis, so you have nothing to lose.

30. A qualified physical therapist will be able to give you a safe workout routine that will help you feel better and lesson the severity of your arthritis symptoms. Take your time in learning the exercises suitable for your needs, including exercises in warming up and cooling down; this will allow you to exercise to your limits without risking injury. Exercise will help arthritis sufferers in a multitude of ways. It strengthens the body and enables the affected joints to still remain in use, instead of being left to languish.

31. While yoga may not have a wealth of research and evidence in regards to its effectiveness for dealing with arthritis, it is often recommended. Yoga involves stretching, full body conditioning and allows for group interaction which is great for stresses involved with arthritis. Use yoga not only for your body therapy but also for your mental well-being as well.

32. You want your arthritis treatment to stop pain and stiffness at their source while also preventing additional damage. Just looking for pain treatment could result in further issues than what you are already encountering, and you could just be pacifying your condition while allowing it to progress further.

33. Protein should be a key part of your diet, when battling arthritis fatigue. You need protein to rebuild the parts of your body which are damaged by exercise or injury, so ensuring that you get an ample amount in your diet is hugely important. If you don't like to eat meat, try adding some protein powder to a smoothie for breakfast.

34. Take a moment to relax on occasion. If you are out being active, you may be hindered by your arthritis. Take occasional breaks so that your body can enjoy peaceful moments while it regains energy.

35. Stay away from heating pads if your arthritis is flaring up. All they are going to do is make your symptoms worse. Instead, apply a cold compress to the area where your arthritis is located. You could even wrap a package of frozen peas or

another frozen vegetable in a towel and apply to the area.

36. Make sure you have a stretching regimen. One of the main problems a sufferer of arthritis has to go through is losing how flexible they are. Losing flexibility can be slowed or even prevented if you take the time to stretch every muscle on a daily basis. Begin at the bottom, with the feet, and slowly make your way up your body to give yourself a total stretch.

37. Investing in a home sauna might just help to alleviate your arthritis pain. The combination of heat and moisture in the sauna can reduce the inflammation, therby reducing the pain. You need to go to the sauna regularly to see results.

38. Have a regular eating schedule. Test your body to find out what eating pattern works best for you, and set up a distinct schedule around those times. If you find yourself hungry at a time when you are not scheduled to eat, have a light nutritious snack to keep yourself energetic and on schedule.

39. You need to shed pounds. Carrying around excess weight can lead to swollen and inflamed conditions when you have arthritis. Too much

weight causes more joint strain, and that is what causes the painful flareups. Losing weight will take a lot of pressure off your joints.

40. Eat foods that are rich in vitamin C to promote healthier joints and reduce pain from arthritis. Vitamin C is proven to offer an essential vitamin that promotes joint health and can reduce the effects of arthritis and damage of joints. You can fill your diet with tasty treats like oranges and grapefruit to reduce your pain and joint damage effectively and naturally.

41. Stay active by taking a walk every evening for 20 minutes. You aren't trying to speed walk or run a marathon, you just need to keep your body in the habit of moving regularly and working out any stiffness in your joints. Regular walks will go a long way towards tempering your arthritis symptoms.

42. Add Epsom salt to your bath water. Epsom salts relax the body and help relieve stiffness, swelling, and pain. Combining these great benefits with a warm bath in the morning hours can easily increase flexibility and reduce pain, allowing you to have a more energized and relaxed day ahead of you.

43. If you are going to be doing a lot of prep work in the kitchen, save your joints by sitting at a table instead of standing at your counter. Spending too much time in the same standing position can put a lot of unnecessary stress on your joints that you will regret later. Get a portable cutting board and take a seat at the table.

44. If your arthritis causes pain and stiffness, try rubbing Castor oil into the affected areas. The oil has therapeutic properties, and the act of massage also helps. A great massage will increase the blood flow to areas where you are experiencing pain, and the castor oil will relieve stiffness.

45. Find a rubber mat to place at your stove to help prevent back and leg pain while you are standing and cooking. These buoyancy of these mats help keep pressure off of your legs which will do wonders for keeping your body feeling healthy. Buy one as well for in front of your sink to use when you are washing dishes.

46. When making a new purchase for your home or kitchen, keep your arthritis in mind when you are deciding what to buy. Buy items that are lightweight and that don't require repetitive

movements. Just simply buying an electric can opener can save your hands from a lot of pain and stress.

47. Arthritis comes in three different types and they are psoriatic arthritis, osteoarthritis and rheumatoid arthritis. Each of these arthritis conditions have their own ideal treatment.

48. Many people have found heat and cold treatments to be very good therapy for arthritis. Try using an old pure cotton sock filled with dry rice as an easy, mess-free method of applying either heat or cold. Put it in a plastic bag in the freezer to prepare for cold therapy. Pop it in the microwave briefly to prepare it for heat therapy.

49. Some studies have proven that weight training can reduce arthritis pain by increasing and maintaining muscle strength. Moderate to more high intensity strength training can improve your physical well-being, emotional condition and functionality over the long run. While strength training doesn't produce overnight results that help with your arthritis, when you employ it long term, it can have very positive results.

50. A great way to soothe the pain of arthritis symptoms is to get a massage. If the pain is not

too severe, massages are a great way to help with pain as long as your muscles are not too tender. Massage helps release tension associated with joint stress. Try to find a massage therapist who is familiar with patients who suffer from rheumatoid arthritis.

51. It is helpful to keep a pain diary. Note when and how you experience the pain, its severity, and what you're doing to ease it. You should record what medications you take, if you skip it and other key info. This sort of information will help your physician tackle your condition.

52. It is important that you try not to put too much stress on your joints if you suffer from arthritis. The only thing that this is going to do is make your arthritis worse. Instead, be sure that you don't overdo it when you have to use your arms or legs for an activity.

53. If you suffer from arthritis, try not to wear clothing that is too tight against your skin. Tight clothing is just going to put more pressure on your joints, which in turn, will increase your pain. Instead, try to wear clothes that have enough room in them so that you are comfortable.

54. Buy products that are specially designed for arthritis sufferers. There is no need to struggle with tasks like opening a jar, buttoning your shirt or turning a doorknob when there are products on the market designed to help you do all of those things. In fact, there are products designed to help arthritis sufferers with just about any task you can think of. Try searching online for arthritis-friendly products or check with any of the leading arthritis organizations for a list of helpful products.

55. Exercising can help you manage your arthritis symptoms by helping you to lose weight. Weight loss can help your joints function more efficiently and help keep those symptoms under control. Talk with your doctor about setting up an exercise plan that you can do safely on a routine basis.

56. Check with your doctor before starting a vitamin regimen. There are multiple conflicting studies associated with different vitamins, so you want to make sure you are taking the ones that will be most beneficial to you. Your doctor will be able to tell you which vitamins are best for your body, as well as how often you should take them.

57. Be sure you understand what the symptoms of arthritis are. A great thing to do for your arthritis is diagnose it early, so you should learn all the symptoms and signs you will have. If you recognize the first symptoms when they occur, you can consult a doctor, get your issue diagnosed, and get started on a treatment plan at the earliest, most effective time.

58. Find a health care professional that you trust and are comfortable speaking with. Arthritis sufferers need to make frequent visits to the doctor to treat painful issues and get regular check ups. If you are not comfortable with your physician, you may not be entirely truthful or trusting of them, so find one that you enjoy working with.

59. Use gardening as an effective therapy against arthritis. There are so many studies out there about arthritis, natural therapies, and one of the top therapies identified is gardening. Simply planting a small garden in your backyard or gardening with some pals can be such a great help in relaxation and relief of your pain.

60. Celebrate the small stuff! Arthritis can slow you down! If you were unable to get to your mailbox six months ago, and now you can, throw yourself

a little celebration! Keeping yourself happy and positive can help you and others see that you are not a helpless creature, and that you are working hard to reach your goals! Don't stop!

61. Keep others aware of what's going on with you. Inform your friends and loved ones about the nature of arthritis and how the disease manifests itself. It's possible that arthritis can change who you once were by affecting your mood or character, which can confuse those who care about you. Let others understand what you're going through so they can offer more help.

62. After you are done with dinner, go for a walk. If you take a walk after supper on a regular basis, you may feel better and have increased energy during the remainder of the evening. Taking a walk with family members or friends, in addition to improving your health, allows you to spend time with people you care about.

63. Ask your doctor for copies of their notes. Having a copy of what they have written about you will allow you to point out any flaws or mistakes, as well as clarify what the doctor may believe to be aggravating symptoms. Most doctors will readily hand these to you, so that you can examine them as well.

64. Carry less. Having arthritis in the shoulders is more common than you think, especially in women. Carrying large shoulder or messenger bags can cause both neck and shoulder inflammation and swelling. If you have to carry a bag, it should be light.

65. Keep a diary for your sake and review, as well as bringing it to your doctor's visits. Your doctor will then be able to tell how you are doing without making you think you have to have total recall of all events. The diary also keeps track of different practices you have incorporated and their effects.

66. Arthritis is a debilitating disease that causes inflammation of the joints, but there are many ways to treat it. One possible arthritis treatment with a long history, though it is less common today, is urtication, or beating with nettles. It is a natural form of therapy that is effective with all types of arthritis.

67. When you are diagnosed with arthritis, your doctor will give you a treatment plan which will incorporate many different things, including diet and exercise. It is important to familiarize yourself with this plan and implement it daily. As

you do, there will be things you will add to the plan or things that will change according to what your body needs.

68. Create a support system that includes other patients with arthritis. Friends and family members may not always be supportive of the pain you're in, or may simply not understand the crippling nature of the condition. Having friends with arthritis can give you someone to talk to about your pain, who understands the problem and won't judge you, while also taking the stress off of your family, when trying to deal with your issues.

69. Exercise is one of the best medicines for arthritis. It is a great help in reducing pain and stiffness in your joints. It will increase your flexibility and the strength of your muscles which will help your body avoid further injury. Make sure to make time every day for exercise and you will see the benefits.

70. Cigarettes have been blamed for diminished flexibility and could cause arthritis flare-ups. Quitting smoking may be difficult, but it is much easier to put down a cigarette when you are aware of the negative effects that it has on your arthritis.

71. A daily routine of stretching your muscles is one of the best things to start. One of the most common complaints associated with arthritis is an overall loss of muscle and joint elasticity. By establishing a routine to stretch on a regular basis, you can help delay or completely prevent loss in your flexibility. Start with your feet, and move upwards across your body all the way to your head.

72. Take a warm morning shower. Many people who suffer from arthritis have the stiffest joints when they wake up. Starting your day off with a warm shower will loosen your joints enough that you should be able to stretch them, which will help to prevent any stiffness you may experience later in the day.

73. Take advantage of physical therapy. A physical therapist helps you develop an exercise routine that will increase your flexibility. Follow their directions to a tee, and you will be able to get your life back to normal.

74. Have a regular eating schedule. Test your body to find out what eating pattern works best for you, and set up a distinct schedule around those times. If you find yourself hungry at a time when

you are not scheduled to eat, have a light nutritious snack to keep yourself energetic and on schedule.

75. Take a walk after dinner. Walking after dinner will increase your energy levels and improve the way you feel, both physically and emotionally. Even a quick walk with a pal will offer numerous health benefits and opportunities to spend quality time together.

76. To help relieve your pain and joint stiffness, you can rub them with castor oil. While the oil itself has many positive benefits for your joints, massaging it in can actually give you double the relief. The act of massaging increases circulation in the area and will work to reduce swelling, and the oil will get to work on your stiffness.

77. You may benefit from participating in a yoga class that will positively effect your overall health if you have arthritis. It has mental benefits in addition to making you feel great physically, and both are important to helping you cope with the symptoms. If you do not want to join a public class, there are a number of yoga DVDs on the market. Working out along with a DVD allows you to get the same benefit without having to leave the comfort of your home.

78. Sleep rests your joints and restores your body's energy so that you are able to handle pain. If you do not get the proper amount of sleep, then you are not equipped to deal with arthritis. If you feel rather tired throughout the day, take a nap in order to replenish your energy level as well.

79. When dealing with arthritis pain you have to protect your joints. Always be thinking about your joints and your joint health and protect them from injury. So be careful; instead of lifting a heavy object, slide it, or use your shoulder to open a door instead of using your hand.

80. Sometimes, the treatments that your doctor offers for arthritis can be assisted and enhanced with alternative treatments such as hydrotherapy, yoga, hot and cold therapy or some herbal or dietary supplements. Be sure to ask your doctor about alternative treatments that will help you make the most of your arthritis care.

81. One good treatment for arthritis pain is LED light therapy. LED devices do not cost much, they are easy to use, and could significantly reduce the pain from arthritis. You can find these useful devices in your neighborhood drug store or discount store. If you use LED therapy

for 15 to 30 minutes two times every day, you can lesson your arthritic pain.

82. Some people use hot wax for pain relief from arthritis. Bathing arthritic hands and feet in hot wax has been shown to ease the pain and inflammation that arthritis can create. A hot wax treatment has the same advantage as a soak in a warm tub. The wax will surround your joints completely and provide pain relief from every angle.

83. Don't push yourself too hard when you're dealing with arthritis; cut back your schedule of household chores. Partition your cleaning routine into single jobs that can be completed one per day.

84. Maintain the right posture all the time. Though proper nutrition and fitness are important, you may be surprised to learn that posture will affect arthritic conditions in a large way. Keep your back straight as you sit up, and keep your feet twelve inches apart from each other. If you maintain good posture, it helps reduce the stress on your joints, which then reduces your pain.

85. You want to practice yoga or meditation if you suffer from chronic arthritis. Relaxing your body

is what these things will do for you, and it can help you better deal with the symptoms associated with arthritis. Ideal practice time for these techniques is three or four times a week.

86. To use a manual stapler while living with arthritis, press down on the stapler with your forearm. Do this instead of using your wrist. The wrist is one area that can become especially sensitive and painful during an arthritis flare up. Keeping from having to use it during those moments means less pain for you, and the task getting accomplished faster too.

87. Newly constructed homes can be modified to make living with your arthritis more manageable. Your builder or contractor will be happy to sit down and come up with ideas with you. Completing small modifications such as these can ease your pain and make your life easier.

88. If you find that your arthritis is getting worse and you cannot figure out why, you want to tell your doctors about certain medications that you are taking. Believe it or not, one of the side effects of many common medications is arthritis flare ups, and if this is the case for you, your doctor may have to switch your medication.

89. Get the proper amount of exercise, and make sure it is the right kind. Exercise will improve your state of mind at the same time that it keeps you healthy, fit, and flexible. Performing low impact exercises will prevent inflammation of your joints, but make sure you never overdo it. Pain is a clear indication that you need to take a break.

90. Take a warm morning shower. Many people who suffer from arthritis have the stiffest joints when they wake up. Starting your day off with a warm shower will loosen your joints enough that you should be able to stretch them, which will help to prevent any stiffness you may experience later in the day.

91. Get support from others who are dealing with psoriatic arthritis. The fatigue that is caused by this condition can make you feel closed off from the world. Do not make the mistake of drawing into yourself and thinking no one understands you. Joining a support group can do wonders for helping you accept your condition and find ways around your new energy levels.

92. When used with a combination of medicines and other treatments, hypnosis has been proven to help with arthritis. Although doctors are not

sure why, patient studies have shown that hypnosis can ease arthritis pain in up to 75% of patients. It is recommended that patients have three rounds of hypnotherapy for the most effective results.

93. For those that have arthritis in their knees, Hyaluronic acid injections are a great option. Because people who have arthritis in their knees are lacking lubrication to keep their joints in top condition, these injections are a great way to give knees lubrication. Speak with your doctor before taking these injections.

94. If you are going to perform any strenuous activity, make sure to utilize assistant devices. If you are planning an activity that involves lifting or reaching or even if you have a lot of writing to do which causes pain in your hands, consider whether there are devices or alternatives that will make these activities less painful for you to engage in them. An increase in damage will also mean in increase in pain, so it's best to not put pressure on your joints to begin with.

95. Use light exercises and stretching to prevent further joint damage and pain from arthritis. light exercise avoids excess strain on the joints and you will find that it creates more limber and

flexible joints that are conditioned for healthier activity. With stretching, you are giving yourself more flexibility for common activities you will encounter without causing pain from inflamed joints.

96. Do not be afraid to consider surgery. Many people who suffer with arthritis will initially balk at the thought of having surgery done to correct an issue. Let your doctor coach you on what may be the best method of treatment for you, and if surgery is an effective option, try not to immediately dismiss it.

97. Counseling may be able to help you better deal with the emotions you are experiencing about arthritis. Chronic physical pain is often accompanied by feelings of being overwhelmed by the disease. Talk to a counselor to help you deal with the emotions in the best way possible.

98. Occupational therapy has been known to help people who suffer from arthritis. Sometimes this kind of therapy is covered by many health insurance plans. Occupational therapy will help identify problem areas in your lifestyle and work with you to find ways to eliminate them or help you work with them to lead a more pain free life.

99. Try including Mediterranean food in your diet. A study came out several years ago that found that arthritis sufferers who consistently ate Mediterranean fruits, vegetables, cereals and olive oil over a period of three months had better daily functioning that other patients. Since eating more fruits and vegetables is good for your health anyway, it is definitely worth a try.

100. If you suffer from the pain of arthritis flare ups, try to remember to keep your pain relievers handy. Many pain relievers like ibuprofen can help relieve symptoms of arthritis flare ups in as little as 15 minutes. So make sure to keep a bottle of your most effective pain reliever close at hand.

101. Learn as much as you can about the disease. The more you know about the symptoms and treatments for arthritis, the more of an active role you can play in your treatment plan. It can also help you to feel less alone, to read about what others with the condition are going through and what they've been trying.

102. Make sure you don't smoke. Smoking has been shown to increase your risk of developing rheumatoid arthritis. Not only that, but if you do develop it, smoking has been shown to worsen the joint damage. Patients who smoke most

often have much more severe symptoms than those patients who don't smoke.

103.   Lay on your thigh, along with pressing it down using your hand. This eliminates the need to grip with aching fingers.

104.   In order to have the energy you need to cope with your arthritis symptoms, it is important to get plenty of sleep. Dealing with the pain and inflammation of arthritis can take a toll on your body and leave you feeling fatigued. The best way to keep your energy up is by making sure you are getting enough sleep. If you have trouble sleeping, try eliminating caffeine or talk to your doctor about medications that may help.

105.   Your best bet is to seek out a physical therapist to work with. A professional can establish an efficient workout routine to help you deal with pain on a daily basis and reduce the swelling. Follow this plan religiously, and you will start to feel positive results.

106.   When used with a combination of medicines and other treatments, hypnosis has been proven to help with arthritis. Although doctors are not sure why, patient studies have shown that hypnosis can ease arthritis pain in up to 75% of

patients. It is recommended that patients have three rounds of hypnotherapy for the most effective results.

107. Get a professional massage. Having a massage done by someone who specializes in arthritis pain can be a delightful treat to any sufferer. These experienced professionals know how to target painful spots and work out tension and pressure that may be hindering your flexibility. If you cannot afford this, have a family member look up techniques and try them out.

108. Communicate and share your arthritis problem with your family and friends. They might be able to help you with certain tasks or simply provide you with the support you need. If you tell your support system what kind of pain you are experiencing, they will let you slide.

109. Let the sun in. Vitamin D has been shown to help relieve some symptoms of arthritis, and sunshine is well-known for increasing positive thoughts and bettering moods. Opening your blinds for around fifteen minutes every day can be enough to give you some great benefits, while still being in the comfort of your home.

110.   Watch your knees. Your knees absorb at least three times the impact of any other joint on your body, so they need extra care. Always make sure to use pads when kneeling and try to flex them often. Sitting cross-legged for too long can also cause issues, so you should stretch them out on a regular basis.

111.   Do not be afraid to consider surgery. Many people who suffer with arthritis will initially balk at the thought of having surgery done to correct an issue. Let your doctor coach you on what may be the best method of treatment for you, and if surgery is an effective option, try not to immediately dismiss it.

112.   Watch for symptoms of depression when you are dealing with psoriatic arthritis. The fatigue you experience with psoriatic arthritis can mask the symptoms of depression. It is hard to feel like you will ever be normal again after the diagnosis. Make sure to see a doctor and deal with symptoms of depression.

113.   It used to be common advice to arthritis sufferers to avoid consuming alcoholic beverages. Studies reveal that moderate alcohol consumption does not have any adverse effects on people who have arthritis. There is even

evidence that moderate consumption of alcohol can reduce the symptoms of arthritis.

114.   Stop smoking. Smoking not only increase the chances of getting arthritis, it also causes the sufferer to have more painful symptoms and more damage to their joints than those who do not smoke. Of course, there are a variety of other health benefits that are associated with not smoking as well, so it is important to make a change as soon as possible.

115.   Do not be uncomfortable about asking for help or finding someone who can help you in times of discomfort just by being there or giving you an ear to listen to. Having a support system of close friends or family will help you take some of the worry and stress out of your daily routine just by being able to talk or have a shoulder to lean on.

116.   When kitchen work starts making you feel a little unsteady on your feet, take the stress off of arthritic joints with a stable, light-weight kitchen stool. Keeping a basic four-legged stool in the kitchen can get you off of your feet and still allow you to sit at a comfortable height for work on counters or the stove top.

117.   Try focused relaxation as a means of fighting the fatigue often associated with the affects of arthritis. Some effective ideas that can relieve your stress and reinvigorate your body include meditating, taking a hot bath or shower, doing some yoga, or practicing deep breathing techniques. Relaxing even for a couple minutes will give you a burst of strength and energy to get you through the rest of your day.

118.   People with arthritis are dealing with both chronic pain and chronic fatigue. Set priorities for your day and stick to them. There will only be so much you can accomplish on a bad day. Figure out what's most important and focus on getting that done, instead of trying to fight the pain and fatigue and do everything anyway.

119.   Try keeping a journal or how arthritis affects your living. This written record will help you understand what in your life is triggering the arthritis. It helps for you to know which methods to use to treat your condition. An added benefit is that the information can easily be shared with your physician, and they can then determine the best course of treatment for you. The journal is a very valuable tool and a good idea all the way around.

120.   Keeping an arthritis journal can actually help you control your symptoms. Each time your arthritis is bothering you, write about what you do that day in your journal. This way, you can start to see a pattern as to what is causing your arthritis pain so you can slow down on that activity.

121.   Exercise is one of the best medicines for arthritis. It is a great help in reducing pain and stiffness in your joints. It will increase your flexibility and the strength of your muscles which will help your body avoid further injury. Make sure to make time every day for exercise and you will see the benefits.

122.   Take a warm morning shower. Many people who suffer from arthritis have the stiffest joints when they wake up. Starting your day off with a warm shower will loosen your joints enough that you should be able to stretch them, which will help to prevent any stiffness you may experience later in the day.

123.   Take the time to plan ahead. Your arthritis could reignite without warning, so to prevent problems, keep a plan ready to be placed into action. Try to plan your jobs to be performed in

sections so you can rest when you need to, and also be able to walk away any time.

124.   Never think bad about yourself, or let others. You might not be comfortable doing specific tasks when you've got arthritis. Guilt and pressure from others will make you feel even worse, so don't let others get you down. Your limitations are no reason to feel like less of a person.

125.   Eat nutritious snacks. Having protein bars, shakes, or fruit can give you the energy your body needs without forcing you to feel like you overate or ruined your health. Choosing healthy snacks will give you the best nutrients to keep your body healthy and strong, which is necessary for anyone with arthritis.

126.   Wear sun block, and protect yourself from UV rays. Those with arthritis are more susceptible to various conditions caused by the sun, including Lupus. Always take the time to cover yourself when you are going to be outdoors or in the sun in order to keep yourself protected.

127.   Try to laugh a lot. Try joking around with your friends, reading a funny book, or watching a

comedy to bring your mood up to lessen stress levels. Laughter is a strong assistant when it comes to people with arthritis, so be sure to use it well and often for the most benefits.

128.   Let the sun in. Vitamin D has been shown to help relieve some symptoms of arthritis, and sunshine is well-known for increasing positive thoughts and bettering moods. Opening your blinds for around fifteen minutes every day can be enough to give you some great benefits, while still being in the comfort of your home.

129.   Be patient with your doctor. With over a hundred different kinds of arthritis in existence, it may take a lot of time and tests before your doctor can tell you which specific one you have. In the meantime, research arthritis in general to find out what you may be dealing with in the future.

130.   If you're struggling with joint pain and stiffness, try massaging the joints with Castor oil. Using a massaging motion to apply the castor oil can provide relief in two ways. Massaging the affected area works with the castor oil to increase the blood flow which will reduce pain, swelling and stiffness.

131.   Find a rubber mat to place at your stove to help prevent back and leg pain while you are standing and cooking. These buoyancy of these mats help keep pressure off of your legs which will do wonders for keeping your body feeling healthy. Buy one as well for in front of your sink to use when you are washing dishes.

132.   Make an effort to regularly take fish oil supplements. These supplements contain omega-3 fatty acids, which are important in helping to control inflammation in the body. They can also help reduce the risk of cardiovascular disease, giving arthritis patients a wide variety of different health benefits when they consume them.

133.   After being diagnosed with arthritis you should go have your eyes checked. Rheumatoid arthritis can cause complications with your vision and in some cases will lead to blindness. Your eye doctor may suggest using anti-inflammatory eye drops to help decrease symptoms of blurred vision, redness, pain, and light sensitivity.

134.   If you are suffering from severe arthritis pain consider acupuncture. Although there is limited research in regards to acupuncture helping with the symptoms of arthritis, many people do say they feel better using this therapy. Skeptics

believe acupuncture is a placebo, but there is not a downside to just giving it a try if it can help.

135.   Thinking positive thoughts can help you to cope with arthritis pain. It might sound silly, but a strong mind/body connection does exist. If your mind thinks positive, it is difficult for your body to feel negative. Fill your life with happiness and you might just find that your pain quickly diminishes.

136.   Stretch your symptom-free joints every day. A warm shower followed by a gentle stretching routine will cause you to feel looser for the rest of the day. Warm, loose muscles will cause less stress on your joints, which means that you will suffer from fewer flare-ups and less pain throughout your day.

137.   Doing low impact exercises, such as swimming, cycling, and walking can help ease arthritis joint discomfort. Talk to your doctor to make sure you do not exert yourself too much.

138.   Getting enough sleep is important for dealing with arthritis. Without enough sleep, your body will be unable to combat arthritis and its pain. Try sleeping about eight hours nightly,

or ten when stressed. Your body's own healing powers improve substantially with good sleep.

139.   If you have arthritis and exercise is difficult, try aquatic activities and exercise programs. Aquatic therapy carefully practiced in warm water is gentle on the joints and muscles which can be a soothing way to exercise while lessoning the pain of arthritis flare-ups. Ask your doctor if there a warm water therapy program could be helpful for you.

140.   Learn tai-chi. Tai-chi is a mind and body connective technique, that is also a form of light martial arts. Using tai-chi can help to convince yourself your body is not in as much pain as your mind believes. Some arthritis sufferers even claim that the use of this method allows them to use their mind to convince their body they are more flexible.

141.   Take a break, but not for too long. When your body feels tired, it is always trying to tell you something. Relaxing both your body and your mind can give you a much needed rest to allow you to be at your best. Try not to relax too much though, as doing so can actually aggravate symptoms.

142.   Before you can get the proper treatment for arthritis, it is important that you know which type you suffer from! There are treatments, both natural and medical, that may help certain kinds of arthritis while doing nothing for other types. If you are uncertain to which kind you have, ask your doctor.

143.   Electrical stimulation can help to relieve the symptoms of osteoarthritis. This treatment has been proven in reducing arthritic knee swelling and pain simultaneously.

144.   Try acupuncture. While many people believe this method does not really work, studies have shown that using it can actually release pain relieving endorphins. This can work wonders for arthritis sufferers by targeting painful inflammation and swelling points in the joint, and sending these relieving chemicals to the area to trigger immediate relief.

145.   Know how to spot the symptoms of arthritis. Do yourself a favor and get it diagnosed early, as soon as you notice possible symptoms. Talk to a doctor right away if you have any of these symptoms, so that you can be properly diagnosed and develop a treatment plan.

146.   Have a regular eating schedule. Test your body to find out what eating pattern works best for you, and set up a distinct schedule around those times. If you find yourself hungry at a time when you are not scheduled to eat, have a light nutritious snack to keep yourself energetic and on schedule.

147.   Have a positive attitude. Negativity causes stress and depression, both of which can be very harmful to someone suffering from arthritis. Remove negative influences from your life, and learn to see the positive side of anything that happens. Doing so will keep you going for much longer than if you let sadness overcome.

148.   Celebrate the small stuff! Arthritis can slow you down! If you were unable to get to your mailbox six months ago, and now you can, throw yourself a little celebration! Keeping yourself happy and positive can help you and others see that you are not a helpless creature, and that you are working hard to reach your goals! Don't stop!

149.   Always use proper form when you are exercising. Having an improper grip or stance can put massive amounts of stress on your joints, so you should always try to begin exercising at a gym or therapist's office. These professionals can

correct the way you are exercising, and prevent you from causing unnecessary injuries.

150. Never wear tight bandages to help with arthritis pain. Having a tight bandage actually will cause more pain and issues, because you are effectively reducing blood flow to the area. This will cause more swelling and stiffness when the bandage is eventually removed, and can even cause permanent damage if left on too long.

151. Document your condition in a diary. This may help you and your doctor determine a proper course of treatment by pinpointing trends which trigger your pain. Write down everything pertinent, such as how much discomfort you feel, the time of day, what food you eat, and so on, so that you will be able to identify patterns.

152. For arthritis pain try using hot and cold treatments to help. Apply heat to the area with a heating pad or try chilling out with an ice pack or ice water to help soothe your joints. Alternating hot and cold can help provide some powerful pain relief as well.

153. Buy accessories for your life and your home that make things easier. For example, you can purchase products that make it easier for you to

open doors or take the lids off of jars. If you can increase the ease of your daily life, you'll reduce pain and stress and improve your attitude.

154.   To enhance your ability to sleep through the discomfort of arthritic pain, try soaking in warm bath salts at night. The bath and the warmth of the water will help relax you and provide some relief from your arthritis pain. Bedtime will come much easier once your body is relaxed.

155.   If you are living with arthritis and happen to be designing a brand new home, make certain to ask for builder modifications that will help you. Your builder or contractor will be happy to sit down and come up with ideas with you. These types of modifications can help to alleviate the pain of stretching sore joints and make your day-to-day life easier.

156.   For people who suffer from arthritis in their hands or fingers, try wearing a hand brace. This is especially helpful for those who are on the computer often. These hand braces will help to keep joints in your hands and fingers supported, even when they are being used a lot.

157.   Discover new ways to eliminate stress so you can relax and manage your arthritis. Stress can be

a factor in how your arthritis develops and in how painful it can be. Look for ways to relax such as meditation or yoga. Light, low impact exercise may help reduce stress and also help your pain.

158.   In order to prevent joint stiffness, incorporate low-impact exercises into your day-to-day routine. Doing too much exercise can cause arthritis to flare up. However, light-to-moderate low-impact exercise can help to keep your joints from stiffening up, giving you more freedom of movement. Some exercises you can do to stay limber include walking, swimming, or bicycling.

159.   It is very important that you drink a lot of water and stay away from sugary drinks if you suffer from chronic arthritis. Water helps to improve muscle and joint strength, while sugary drinks like soda make you gain weight, which causes more pressure to be put on your joints.

160.   Make sure your doctor is knowledgeable on the subject of arthritis. Some doctors have had extensive training in the field, and know better and more effective treatments than other doctors might. Ask your doctor how much they know about arthritis, and if they would be comfortable

recommending you to someone more experienced.

161.   Learn good posture. The better your stance, the less stress you put on your joints. Ask your doctor for tips on gaining the best posture you can, and work on it daily as a routine. Once you develop good posture, you will feel less pain in your back and knees, as well as your feet and neck.

162.   If you are suffering from severe arthritis pain consider acupuncture. Although there is limited research in regards to acupuncture helping with the symptoms of arthritis, many people do say they feel better using this therapy. Skeptics believe acupuncture is a placebo, but there is not a downside to just giving it a try if it can help.

163.   Always keep good posture. No matter how much you eat, your posture is what causes further pain. Anytime you are sitting, align your back into a straight position, and when you are standing, make sure you keep your feet separated by roughly 12 inches. Doing these things can improve your posture, which helps to keep joint pain at bay.

164.   Meditation can be highly effective in coping with arthritis. The brain is an often overlooked tool in dealing with disease or debilitating conditions. Through meditation you can condition your mind to work for you. You can achieve relaxed states in which you create mantras that program your thinking in regards to how you deal with pain and stress.

165.   Find a balance between being active and restful. It is very beneficial to take breaks in your daily activity that allow your joints to relax and your mind as well. Avoid to much restful behavior as you can create more pain and stiffness by giving in to the comfort of sitting and relaxing. Achieve a balance that you can be consistent with.

166.   Sign up for counseling. A doctor will help you with the medical aspect of arthritis, but counseling will help you with the psychological aspect. Counseling will help you deal with your stress better and perhaps even with your depression if this is the case as well as help you cope with the chronic pain.

167.   While exercise is important, you should take it easy when your arthritis is flaring up. Exercise keeps your joints flexible; however, it does not

help fight the pain associated with arthritis. You should skip the workout if your joints hurt a lot.

168.   If your body wants you to rest, then give in and take five. Arthritis can be managed if you heed your body's messages, so when it tells you to slow down, slow down.

169.   Getting a massage is recommended if your pain isn't too severe. This will relax your muscles and reduce your level of stress. Be sure to find a massage therapist that is able to properly treat arthritis patients. You should likely wait until the next day if you feel your joints are too sore.

170.   If you're overweight, lose weight to help with your arthritis symptoms. As one might expect, an overweight body applies additional stress to the weight-bearing joints, making arthritic flare-ups more likely and more severe. Weight loss stimulates the body to reduce production of the hormones and chemicals that cause inflammation.

171.   Take your time with major clean up tasks if arthritis is a part of your life. Major cleaning tasks, like mopping and changing bed sheets, put a strain on your body. They involve the use, and sometimes over use, of several different muscles

and joints. Take a break when you can or better yet, ask for help. You don't have to do it all in one day.

172.   Keep a diary about the progress of your condition. This journal gives you assistance in determining which things cause your arthritis to flare up. It can also work to learn what will help control your symptoms. Discuss the information you gather with your physician, so that he or she can suggest the best treatment options. It will help you in many ways.

173.   Arthritis can sometimes cause rashes on the arthritic areas on your body or on your face. If this is the case, you can buy cover up and other make up to hide these rashes. Many arthritis sufferers think that they should stay away from make up, which is not true.

174.   Because arthritis can effect the way that you cook, it is important that you buy the proper cookware and utensils. If you pick any old utensil, you may find that you cannot use it. It is recommended that people with arthritis get lightweight cooking utensils that have easy grips.

175.   Always protect your joints when you are dealing with arthritis. Keep your joints moving

throughout the day and avoid holding them in the same position for too long a period of time. Always consider how to best execute a task to minimize stress to your joints.

176.   Establsih a regular stretching routine. Flexibility is one of the major issues for those living with arthritis. Establishing a daily regimen that targets all your muscles is one of the best ways to stay flexible. Start your stretches with your feet, then move up your body until you get to your neck and head.

177.   If you are suffering arthritis in the knees, consider buying a knee brace. Surgery should always be your last option. The brace will help you determine whether you really need the surgery. You can wear your brace while sleeping, too.

178.   Get extra rest before doing something stressful. No matter what anyone tells you, a stressful event in your life can drain you even more quickly, if you have arthritis. Prepare for these events by sleeping in, taking naps, and perhaps even eating a little extra. Having that boost of energy when you need it, will come in very handy.

179. A healthy diet is a key factor in fighting psoriatic arthritis. Make sure to never skip your meals. Keep your diet a healthy mix of proteins, complex carbs, and unsaturated fats to help your body have enough energy to get through the day. A healthy diet will go a long way towards fighting fatigue, which can aggrevate your arthritis.

180. Purchase an ergonomic knife that is designed to help you cut and slice with ease without putting a strain on your joints. These knives give you better leverage so that you can use your body weight to do your cutting instead of using your joints in a repetitive fashion.

181. Whenever you dwell on something, you just make it worse. It is important in your healing process not to dwell on the bad things but instead dwell on the good things. Remember things that are important to you that you want to focus on, and take your mind off of the pain.

182. One if the big factors that has been linked to arthritis and decreasing your overall health is smoking. Do not smoke. This lifestyle factor has been associated and known to cause severe joint damage when coupled with people who have arthritis. So improve your health and make your joints feel better by not smoking.

183.   Many people with arthritis have found that taking yoga classes and learning how to practice it at home can help with arthritis pain. Yoga emphasizes stretching and whole body well-being. This will help you improve motion and make your joints feel better. The Arthritis Foundation recommends using yoga to help with arthritis.

184.   Be sure to keep yourself in the best physical condition possible. Even though, there is not currently a cure for arthritis, that does not mean there will never be. By maintaining your health and keeping fit, you are keeping yourself ready for that possibility. If-and-when a cure is found, you will be ready to try it successfully!

185.   During periods of non-inflammation and with the permission of your doctor, exercise to build energy and slow the onset of pain. Swimming or exercising in water is great for your joints because the water offers resistance without high strain. Water can also keep you cool thereby acting as a natural soother for pain and discomfort should it set in.

186.   Determine what is causing the most pain and what activities are reducing your pain. If you can

find out the triggers for pain and those things that are soothing the pain or aren't causing inflammation, you can better balance your day and refrain from those activities that are causing you greater stress. This will improve your lifestyle as well, giving you a more healthy feeling from day to day that is pain free and enjoyable.

187.   Always stay positive because it dramatically influences your physical state. If the pain of arthritis is always on your mind, you will feel more of it, and it will make life unbearable. Instead, live life in the moment. Focus on comforting and relaxing thoughts instead of dwelling on the pain.

188.   It might seem hard to do but you should exercise often if you have arthritis. If your joints remain inactive, they will deteriorate faster. It is important to make sure you are doing exercises that increase your flexibility as well. When you have arthritis, flexibility translates into a better range of motion and less pain.

189.   Visit a massage therapist on a regular basis if you suffer from arthritis. The massages that these professionals perform on you will help to make your body relax and ease some of the pain in your joints. It is recommended that you visit a

massage therapist every two weeks if you have arthritis.

190.   Exercising can help you manage your arthritis symptoms by helping you to lose weight. Weight loss can help your joints function more efficiently and help keep those symptoms under control. Talk with your doctor about setting up an exercise plan that you can do safely on a routine basis.

191.   Create a routine for stretching. One of the most common problems for people with arthritis is that they lose flexibility. By establishing a routine to stretch on a regular basis, you can help delay or completely prevent loss in your flexibility. Start off with stretching your feet, and then move in an upwards direction across you entire body until you reach your head.

192.   Do not expect to follow the same schedule you followed before your diagnosis. Some types of arthritis can cause serious fatigue and discomfort, and you need to listen to your body. Rest if you need to, or change your schedule around to do activities at the times during the day that you have more flexibility.

193.   Find the best bed possible in which to sleep. People who suffer from arthritis should talk with their doctors about finding out what is the right kind of bed for someone in this condition. Since each individual is distinct and unique, expert advice is required to get the specific bed best for your own particular arthritic condition and circumstances.

194.   Take monthly visits to your doctor to look for different types of vitamin deficiencies. Being low in certain vitamins or minerals, like vitamin B-12 or iron, can cause havoc for arthritis sufferers. It exacerbates the symptoms. By monitoring these levels and keeping them in check, you can avoid painful flare-ups.

195.   Try to lose some weight. Excess weight can increase swelling and inflammation associated with arthritis. If you are overweight it can but extra strain your your joints, this will cause them to flare. Shedding a little weight may be a good idea because it can have an effect on how bad the pain is and how frequently it pops up.

196.   Learn as much as you can about your condition if you have arthritis. The old adage that knowledge is power is especially true in this case. The more you learn about your form of

arthritis and its treatments, the better chance you have of living a full and active life in spite of your condition.

197.   Castor oil can help with joint pain. The oil has active ingredients that will help your joints, and the act of massaging your joint should make the pain disappear. This pressure can help to accelerate blood flow in your body, and eliminate stiffness and tension.

198.   Always make sure that you are wearing properly fitting footwear that does not bind, pinch or rub your feet to help keep arthritis symptoms at bay. Badly fitting shoes can irritate your joints causing issues that will stay with you for the rest of your life. Have your shoes properly fitted to avoid these issues.

199.   Arthritic knees can be very painful, and it is important to try and take stress off or you knees when you have arthritis. One way to do this is by losing weight if you are overweight. Doing this relieves the pressure off of the joints in your knees and helps out immensely.

200.   Make an appointment with a nutritionist, and talk about some foods that have Omega 6 and Omega 3 fatty acids that will work to reduce any

inflammation. Such a diet can help you from becoming overweight. Increase your knowledge about different foods that can keep arthritis pain at bay.

201.   Studies show that doing strength training exercises can increase your muscle strength, as well as relieve arthritis pain. Stronger muscles can lead to a decrease in joint pain and inflammation. Strength training takes some time to see results and is best thought of as a long-term goal.

202.   You need a network of friends and family you can rely upon when dealing with chronic pain. Go to your doctor regularly and keep track of how your condition is progressing. You should also let your friends and family know exactly what you are dealing with, and try to get support from them.

203.   You need to remain mobile with arthritis so make sure you exercise regularly, however, break it down into smaller time portions. Although it might take a big longer to get your full complement of exercise in, research has shown that the benefits really help to ease your arthritis symptoms. Complete 10 minutes of exercise at least three times a day to get maximum results.

204.   An occupational therapist can help you deal with life after an arthritis diagnosis. If you have a good therapist, they can help you find the things that are hurting your arthritis. You'll enjoy a greater quality of life by following your occupational therapist's advice on problems you can avoid or eliminate.

205.   Watch out for co-morbid condition, especially depression. Arthritis and depression can lock you into a feedback loop: you're tired and in pain, so you can't do the things you love, which makes you more upset. Being upset then leads to symptom flare-ups. If you think you are depressed, speak with your doctor about a referral to a psychiatrist.

206.   For people who suffer from chronic arthritis, be careful when choosing a pet for your family. Remember, if your arthritis is acting up or even gets worse, it may be hard for you to care for your pet. Instead, you may want to consider getting a pet that is easier to take care, such as a fish.

207.   Eat the right supplements. Omega 3 fish oils have been shown to greatly reduce inflammation and swelling of joints, as well as help to increase

flexibility. Make sure you are taking these supplements as they are prescribed, and you will quickly find yourself able to do the tasks you were worried you would not be able to do.

208.   Implement a cane into your daily routine for support. Many people equate canes to disability; however, this is not true. If you have less pain when you use a cane you should do it. You may be more receptive to the idea of using a cane if you purchase one that is well-made or unique.

209.   When you have arthritis, you will want to maximize the amount of sleep that you get during the night. If you suffer from arthritis, you need proper rest. During sleep, your body rejuvenates itself and restores energy that your body will need to properly function tomorrow. Try to sleep in complete darkness, switching your clock around, turning off the cellphone, and trying relaxing techniques prior to slumber.

210.   Never forget to protect yourself from UV rays through sunblock and other methods. Get as little sun exposure as you can, as the sun affects almost every sufferer of Lupus. Make sure you cover up and take extra care of yourself while in the sun. You don't want to come up with any more illnesses in the near future when

you have enough of a hard time dealing with arthritis.

211. Stay active by taking a walk every evening for 20 minutes. You aren't trying to speed walk or run a marathon, you just need to keep your body in the habit of moving regularly and working out any stiffness in your joints. Regular walks will go a long way towards tempering your arthritis symptoms.

212. Keep a diary. By keeping track of your daily activities and how much pain you feel, you will be able to find patterns that can help you identify triggers. For your diary to be effective, it should include as much information as possible. Some of the things you should definitely include are the exact date and time you felt pain, where you were, what you were doing, and your most recent meal.

213. Sometimes, the treatments that your doctor offers for arthritis can be assisted and enhanced with alternative treatments such as hydrotherapy, yoga, hot and cold therapy or some herbal or dietary supplements. Be sure to ask your doctor about alternative treatments that will help you make the most of your arthritis care.

214.	Arthritis sufferers have traditionally been advised not to drink alcohol. Studies reveal that moderate alcohol consumption does not have any adverse effects on people who have arthritis. Some studies even suggest that alcohol consumption in moderation may help reduce arthritis symptoms.

215.	If you are suffering from severe arthritis pain consider acupuncture. Although there is limited research in regards to acupuncture helping with the symptoms of arthritis, many people do say they feel better using this therapy. Skeptics believe acupuncture is a placebo, but there is not a downside to just giving it a try if it can help.

216.	Find out more about your condition. Doctors usually know what they are doing, but you can face this condition better if you educate yourself about it. You should find out what causes your arthritis and look for things you can do to ease the pain or improve your condition, that your doctor might not know about.

217.	Get your beauty sleep, even if you have to nap in the afternoon. Be committed to obtaining the rest you need for dealing with pain from arthritis, even it you have to set a clock for naps and breaks.

218.   Sometimes walking from one room to another can be extremely painful for people who suffer from arthritis. Do not make your home into an obstacle course and make your paths around the home as easy to navigate as possible. Have someone help you move your furniture so that there are easy paths to get from one room to another.

219.   Arthritis can flare up if you are feeling stressed. The effects of stress take their toll on your body in many ways, including exacerbating the pain and making arthritis progress. Getting involved in a hobby, exercising and practicing meditation can all be effective ways to relive stress. It will also be helpful to avoid stressful decisions whenever possible.

220.   Do not be uncomfortable about asking for help or finding someone who can help you in times of discomfort just by being there or giving you an ear to listen to. Having a support system of close friends or family will help you take some of the worry and stress out of your daily routine just by being able to talk or have a shoulder to lean on.

221.   Protein should be a key part of your diet, when battling arthritis fatigue. You need protein to rebuild the parts of your body which are damaged by exercise or injury, so ensuring that you get an ample amount in your diet is hugely important. If you don't like to eat meat, try adding some protein powder to a smoothie for breakfast.

222.   If you have arthritis, try reducing your caffeine intake. Some people are extremely sensitive to arthritis. In those individuals, reducing the consumption of caffeine can have a positive effect on arthritis symptoms. Reduce the amount of caffeine you consume gradually to best gauge if your results will be positive ones.

223.   Even though it is hard sometimes, exercising frequently is something you should do if you are dealing with arthritis. Joints which are not exercised get fatigued easier, making your arthritis worse. Increasing your flexibility will also help your arthritis by helping you maintain a wide range of motion.

224.   Make time in your day to do the things you love. Increased stress levels can lead to more arthritis flare-ups. If you find time to do the activities you enjoy, you'll improve your mood

and your energy levels. This kind of effect will lead to lasting improvement for your symptoms.

225.   Squeeze tubes are your friends when living with arthritis. Buy them whenever you have the option. Whether it is the mayonnaise or jelly, opening a jar is a difficult task when your hands hurt. Buy a squeeze tube instead and the task will be much easier to accomplish. This means less pain in the kitchen and a more enjoyable day.

226.   It is important that you get the flu shot if you suffer from arthritis. Just like with many other chronic illnesses, arthritis symptoms will get much worse if you get the flu and could even land you in the hospital. The flu shot is a simple shot that you only have to get once a year.

227.   For people who suffer from chronic arthritis, be careful when choosing a pet for your family. Remember, if your arthritis is acting up or even gets worse, it may be hard for you to care for your pet. Instead, you may want to consider getting a pet that is easier to take care, such as a fish.

228.   Go to a physical therapist. A physical therapist can help you to design a daily workout or stretching plan designed to improve your

strength and flexibility and by extension, reduce arthritis-related strain and pain. Follow this plan religiously, and you will start to feel positive results.

229.   One thing you can do for your joint aches and pains is to give yourself a break with a vacation or some simple time off at home. You want rest and a lot of it, and the best way to stock up on good old rest is by taking that vacation you have always dreamed of, or even by just taking the phone off the hook and laying in bed for a couple days. This gives your joints relief from your daily routine of constantly going.

230.   Ask your doctor for copies of their notes. Having a copy of what they have written about you will allow you to point out any flaws or mistakes, as well as clarify what the doctor may believe to be aggravating symptoms. Most doctors will readily hand these to you, so that you can examine them as well.

231.   Always make sure that you are wearing properly fitting footwear that does not bind, pinch or rub your feet to help keep arthritis symptoms at bay. Badly fitting shoes can irritate your joints causing issues that will stay with you

for the rest of your life. Have your shoes properly fitted to avoid these issues.

232.   Use either hot or cold compresses on your aching joints. This can help to relieve the pain you are feeling. Alternating between hot and cold is also a great way to help your joints feel better. It is important to speak with your doctor about the best way to use this technique.

233.   Try changing your diet to vegetarian or vegan to help with arthritis pain. It is not uncommon for vegetarians with arthritis to report experiencing less pain and stiffness. The antioxidants in green vegetable are said to protect the body from arthritis pain.

234.   Be sure to get regular exercise as part of your arthritis therapy. Avoid exercise that stresses your joints, such as aerobics, running, and possibly, bicycling. Instead, try water aerobics, swimming, and possibly, yoga. These forms of exercise minimize pressure on the joints and maximize flexibility. Remember not to overdo exercise. Give your body ample time to rest and recover.

235.   Sometimes people who suffer from rheumatoid arthritis find it beneficial to get

involved in an active community of other people who also have the condition. Even if you just read blogs and articles written by others who suffer from rheumatoid arthritis, you will feel less isolated and feel more empowered with the knowledge.

236.   You cannot plan when your arthritis will flare, so plan your activities accordingly. If you prepare and plan for arthritis problems before they happen, you will not be disappointed if symptoms show and you have to take a break. If you start an activity, try to make sure you can end at any point so that if you have an arthritis flare up, you can come back to it later.

237.   While yoga may not have a wealth of research and evidence in regards to its effectiveness for dealing with arthritis, it is often recommended. Yoga involves stretching, full body conditioning and allows for group interaction which is great for stresses involved with arthritis. Use yoga not only for your body therapy but also for your mental well-being as well.

238.   Learn as much as you can about the disease. The more you know about the symptoms and treatments for arthritis, the more of an active

role you can play in your treatment plan. It can also help you to feel less alone, to read about what others with the condition are going through and what they've been trying.

239.   For arthritis sufferers, it is important to lose weight if you are overweight or obese. Excess weight just puts more strain and pressure on your arthritic joints, which can make your arthritis even worse. It is a proven fact that every pound you lose is four less pounds of pressure on your knees.

240.   Before you begin self-treating for arthritis pain, be absolutely certain that the cause of your joint pain and stiffness is really osteoarthritis. A lot of people make assumptions that aches and pains they suffer as they age are from arthritis, but a wide variety of ailments can cause joint pain. A CT-Scan is the best way to know if your pain is really caused by arthritis.

241.   It is important that you have enough calcium in your diet if you suffer from arthritis. Medical research has proven that inflammatory arthritis conditions are worse if a person does not have enough calcium in their diet. You can find calcium in many different foods, including milk, cheese, and ice cream.

242.   For people who suffer from arthritis in their hands or fingers, try wearing a hand brace. This is especially helpful for those who are on the computer often. These hand braces will help to keep joints in your hands and fingers supported, even when they are being used a lot.

243.   Make sure to educate yourself as much as possible about rheumatoid arthritis, and how it can affect pregnancy and breastfeeding. There's a lot of different information out there, and being well educated can make all the difference in the world in how you handle your symptoms and flare ups.

244.   Instead of dwelling on the activities you can't do with with your children if you suffer from rheumatoid arthritis, spend time finding things that you can do together. Just because you can't go running around the park with them, doesn't make you a bad parent. Take them to the pool or read stories together. The most important thing is that you spend time together, not how you spend it.

245.   Do not discount the need to get enough sleep when dealing with psoriatic arthritis. You need sleep now even more than before. If you

are having trouble sleeping, talk with your doctor about medications that can help. Keep your bedroom a place for resting so that your body knows that heading to bed means time for sleep.

246.   Eat nutritious snacks. Having protein bars, shakes, or fruit can give you the energy your body needs without forcing you to feel like you overate or ruined your health. Choosing healthy snacks will give you the best nutrients to keep your body healthy and strong, which is necessary for anyone with arthritis.

247.   It is essential that you talk to a physician when your symptoms start appearing and that you begin treatment right away if you need it. The sooner you start treating your arthritis, the less damage you will do to your joints. The most beneficial way to start treatment is to get advice from a doctor early so you can start the treatment when a diagnosis is reached.

248.   Know your limits. Pushing yourself too hard can be detrimental to your health and safety. If you want to attempt something that may be a reach, try to have someone nearby in case you need assistance. You do not want to cause undue stress on your mind or your joints, so give yourself boundaries.

249.   Be sure to share your circumstances with others. Make them aware of how arthritis affects your life. Arthritis will cause moments of frustration, pain and even sour mood in your life, which are all points where those around you will start wondering what is going on. Sharing your arthritis struggles with the people close to you could lead to a stronger support system, and an exchange of vital information.

250.   Put castor oil on your joints in order to lower your pain and stiffness. The massaging action is relaxing and the castor oil is good for the joints. Castor oil relieves some stiffness, while massaging gets blood flowing into the joints, which relieves swelling and pain.

251.   One way to deal with arthritis is to make sure you are coping with it in a positive manner. Focus on wellness and not on sickness. It is not easy when you are in pain to think in a positive way, but you can do it! It will help you and your pain.

252.   New studies have shown that eating foods high in omega-3s will help with arthritis. If you are not a fan of fish and seafood, then you can still reap the benefits of omega-3s by taking a

daily fish oil supplement. It has an additional benefit for helping people who are high risk for cardiovascular disease as well.

253.   When you are thinking about looking into herbal treatments to help you treat your arthritis symptoms, keep in mind that herbal remedies are not regulated by the FDA. You should always seek the advice of your physician and/or a skilled and experienced herbalist when considering the use of herbal remedies.

254.   Make sure you have appropriate footwear if you are going to be working out. Worn out shoes distribute your weight unevenly. As a result, you will feel more pain in your legs. It is essential to replace workout shoes as soon as you notice that the bottom of your shoes has become uneven to make sure you get the best results.

255.   If you have rheumatoid arthritis, keep a journal. Analyzing these writings will help you to identify the causes of your flare-ups. Understanding the root of the problem is the first step towards improving your condition. You can share this information with your doctor to help him best prescribe treatment options. It is a helpful tool for many purposes.

256.   Always stick to your physical therapy regimen. Arthritis takes a mental toll on a person. It limits their options in life, and therapy can help them realize that they are not alone and helpless. Arthritis sufferers also are more likely to develop conditions like depression, so going to therapy, whether individual or group, can address these important concerns.

257.   Take a break, but not for too long. When your body feels tired, it is always trying to tell you something. Relaxing both your body and your mind can give you a much needed rest to allow you to be at your best. Try not to relax too much though, as doing so can actually aggravate symptoms.

258.   If you suffer from arthritis, it is very important that you do not get too stressed out. Stress makes the body tense, which in turn, makes your arthritis worse. It is important that you keep your body relaxed at all times to prevent your joints from getting too stiff and cramped.

259.   If you have been diagnosed with chronic arthritis, regular visits to a hot sauna may be in order. The wet heat and steam will be helpful in reducing inflammation, and inflammation is a

main cause of the pain. In order to be effective, you have to visit the sauna on a regular basis.

260.   Have a positive attitude. Negativity causes stress and depression, both of which can be very harmful to someone suffering from arthritis. Remove negative influences from your life, and learn to see the positive side of anything that happens. Doing so will keep you going for much longer than if you let sadness overcome.

261.   Get educated about your unique condition. There are over a hundred different types of arthritis, and learning about yours will only help you be able to manage it more effectively. Get a diagnosis from a doctor, and then do your own research to find out what to expect and how to deal with it.

262.   If you are going to be doing a lot of prep work in the kitchen, save your joints by sitting at a table instead of standing at your counter. Spending too much time in the same standing position can put a lot of unnecessary stress on your joints that you will regret later. Get a portable cutting board and take a seat at the table.

263.   Never wear high heels. Women who suffer from arthritis should stay far away from these shoes, as they put extra stress on the ankles and knees. Wearing these can actually cause tears in the tendons surrounding joints, which will only worsen any inflammation and pain that already exists in the area.

264.   Many people tend to have bad posture and do all sorts of things that wreak havoc on their bodies. When you have arthritis, it is even more important to pay close attention to things like this. You need to make sure you maintain good posture and the correct positioning of your body.

265.   Arthritis is simply joint inflammation and it can be treated effectively. All cases of arthritis can be treated through an ancient old set of remedies known as urtication. It's worth trying because it's natural and has been proven to help.

266.   Just because there is no cure for arthritis doesn't mean you can't find relief from the pain. Be sure to pay close attention to your doctor's advice regarding diet, exercise, supplements and pain relievers. By remaining pro-active in your treatment plan you can overcome a great deal of the pain and debilitation of arthritis.

267.   Take preventative steps to prevent your arthritis from worsening. Variations in needs, pain levels, and symptoms are endless due to the millions of patients and hundreds of types of arthritis. You have to know the available treatments and know enough to match the right treatment to your particular arthritis.

268.   If you suffer from arthritis, do your best to use diet and moderate exercise to lose any unnecessary weight you are carrying. Excess weight puts more stress on bones and joints and causes them to wear out more quickly. Losing weight will not only lessen the stress on your back, hips and knees, but also make it easier to engage in more physical exercise.

269.   Many people stop trying to treat themselves, so they give up. There are different kinds of arthritis, and there are different ways to treat it. What is effective for one person may not work for another. You have to keep looking for new treatments, and try them until you eventually find out one that is right for you.

270.   The pain is the major thing that makes arthritis so hard to live with. Learn to manage your pain better so that it affects your life less. The key is to discover the type of arthritis you

have, and learn what treatments are available for that specific affliction.

271.   Avoid exposure to cigarette smoke, yours or anyone else's. The nicotine from cigarettes reduces the blood flow to your extremities which can provide temporary relief. Blood flow reduction can cause damage to your joints and this will make arthritis worse.

272.   If you are suffering from rheumatoid arthritis, make sure you're getting enough omega-3 in your diet. If you're not, consider taking a supplement like fish oil to help get those levels up. Studies have shown that omega-3 has many anti-inflammatory benefits for those who suffer from rheumatoid arthritis.

273.   It is important that you try not to put too much stress on your joints if you suffer from arthritis. The only thing that this is going to do is make your arthritis worse. Instead, be sure that you don't overdo it when you have to use your arms or legs for an activity.

274.   Visit a massage therapist on a regular basis if you suffer from arthritis. The massages that these professionals perform on you will help to make your body relax and ease some of the pain

in your joints. It is recommended that you visit a massage therapist every two weeks if you have arthritis.

275.   If you are a woman who suffers from arthritis in your back, you may want to think about changing what bras you wear. Believe it or not, certain bras can make your arthritis worse by putting pressure on your back. There are actually bras that are made just for women with arthritis.

276.   Make sure to educate yourself as much as possible about rheumatoid arthritis, and how it can affect pregnancy and breastfeeding. There's a lot of different information out there, and being well educated can make all the difference in the world in how you handle your symptoms and flare ups.

277.   Buy your children's clothing with zippers and loose fitting clothing if you are a parent dealing with rheumatoid arthritis. Trying to handle a button or a snap can be a nightmare when you have rheumatoid arthritis. Don't suffer just to get your child the cutest outfit in the store.

278.   Instead of dwelling on the activities you can't do with with your children if you suffer from rheumatoid arthritis, spend time finding things

that you can do together. Just because you can't go running around the park with them, doesn't make you a bad parent. Take them to the pool or read stories together. The most important thing is that you spend time together, not how you spend it.

279.   Get a professional massage. Having a massage done by someone who specializes in arthritis pain can be a delightful treat to any sufferer. These experienced professionals know how to target painful spots and work out tension and pressure that may be hindering your flexibility. If you cannot afford this, have a family member look up techniques and try them out.

280.   Eat nutritious snacks. Having protein bars, shakes, or fruit can give you the energy your body needs without forcing you to feel like you overate or ruined your health. Choosing healthy snacks will give you the best nutrients to keep your body healthy and strong, which is necessary for anyone with arthritis.

281.   Learn the information that is out there about your condition. When you get the diagnosis of your specific type of arthritis, hit the internet and all the sources that are offered, even pamphlets and brochures from the doctor's office, all about

arthritis and your specific type, so you know what you are dealing with and how to fight back.

282.   Laugh often. Stress can be reduced significantly when you watch a humorous film, laugh at jokes or read an entertaining book. Laughter is a great asset to have when you are suffering from arthritis, be sure you use it as much as you can.

283.   Pay close attention to your medical treatment plan. Many arthritis sufferers make the mistake of simply closing their minds to what their doctors are saying to them. A good patient should take notes on what the doctor is telling them, as well as what the pharmacist says. Doing this can keep you informed on your own condition.

284.   Try your best to avoid smoking. When you do, you can minimize some pains that are associated with arthritis, like pain and swelling. There have been studies done on nonsmokers and it shows that they don't have as many problems with pain from arthritis and swollen joints as smokers do. If you do smoke, seriously think about quitting to help with your symptoms. If you are having trouble quitting on your own,

consult with your doctor who can prescribe a medication that will help.

285.   If you are like the typical arthritis sufferer, you are likely trying new treatments and coping methods all the time. Prior to beginning a new treatment, you should rate the current level of your pain you are feeling. This will allow you to find out where your pain is as you're trying new ideas and treatments.

286.   When dealing with arthritis pain you have to protect your joints. Always be thinking about your joints and your joint health and protect them from injury. So be careful; instead of lifting a heavy object, slide it, or use your shoulder to open a door instead of using your hand.

287.   You must remain proactive in the process of creating an arthritis therapy program. Bear in mind that every case of arthritis is different, and that your condition requires its own special treatment plan. You need to understand what treatment options are out there, and which of those would benefit you the most.

288.   Be sure to get enough exercise and that you are doing the right kinds of exercise. People with arthritis should choose exercises that support

and strengthen the joints, such as swimming, instead of exercises that damage them, such as running. Failing to exercise can also increase joint stiffness and pain.

289.   Try different treatments with hot and cold packs to see what works for you. Different patients have different success with hot or cold compresses. Generally, chronic pain responds well to heat, while sudden onset pain responds best to cold packs. Everyone is different, however, and your initial treatment attempts may not bring immediate relief.

290.   Place the clipper on your thigh, and use your palm to press the clipper closed. This avoids using your fingers and facilitates the task.

291.   Cool down your joints and stop physical activity if you start feeling arthritis pain. Rest in a cool environment and use cold packs or mists of cold water to help reduce the pain and swelling caused by injury. Make sure to rest the injured joints and let them have time to get back to fighting order before using them for any difficult tasks.

292.   Take the time to have your family educated about your rheumatoid arthritis and the different

challenges that will occur while you live with this condition. There are classes available through The Arthritis Foundation, and there are many books available that can be used to teach your family about the condition.

293.   Arthritis sufferers can benefit from taking fish oil. Omega-3 fatty acids in fish oils can reduce joint pain. Vitamin and health food stores have many quality brands of fish oil and it is becoming more readily available in grocery stores as well.

294.   Do not be afraid to consider surgery. Many people who suffer with arthritis will initially balk at the thought of having surgery done to correct an issue. Let your doctor coach you on what may be the best method of treatment for you, and if surgery is an effective option, try not to immediately dismiss it.

295.   Ask your doctor for copies of their notes. Having a copy of what they have written about you will allow you to point out any flaws or mistakes, as well as clarify what the doctor may believe to be aggravating symptoms. Most doctors will readily hand these to you, so that you can examine them as well.

296.   Find a hobby that you can easily perform. Many people who suffer from arthritis spend their days wishing they had something they could actually do, and you can prevent this boredom by searching out your own new hobby. Whether it is painting or dancing, having something to get you moving will keep you healthy.

297.   Do not use your hands if you don't have to. Even if they are not currently bothering you, protect them as much as possible; if you can open a door by pushing it with you shoulder, do so. This will help lessen the amount of pain that you feel in your joints and allow you to lead a more regular life.

298.   You cannot plan when your arthritis will flare, so plan your activities accordingly. If you prepare and plan for arthritis problems before they happen, you will not be disappointed if symptoms show and you have to take a break. If you start an activity, try to make sure you can end at any point so that if you have an arthritis flare up, you can come back to it later.

299.   Find out more about your condition. Doctors usually know what they are doing, but you can face this condition better if you educate yourself about it. You should find out what

causes your arthritis and look for things you can do to ease the pain or improve your condition, that your doctor might not know about.

300.   Sometimes walking from one room to another can be extremely painful for people who suffer from arthritis. Do not make your home into an obstacle course and make your paths around the home as easy to navigate as possible. Have someone help you move your furniture so that there are easy paths to get from one room to another.

301.   Determine what is causing the most pain and what activities are reducing your pain. If you can find out the triggers for pain and those things that are soothing the pain or aren't causing inflammation, you can better balance your day and refrain from those activities that are causing you greater stress. This will improve your lifestyle as well, giving you a more healthy feeling from day to day that is pain free and enjoyable.

302.   For women dealing with arthritis pain, put your high heels aside and choose lower heels or supportive flat shoes. Any shoe that stresses the feet is also going to stress the joints, even those in the back. Try to get some running shoes that

provide more support or a pair of orthopedic dress shoes when you're going to work.

303.   Do not be afraid to ask for help when dealing with arthritis pain. Many people are more than willing to help and all you have to do is ask. Maybe a neighbor could deliver your mail for you, or a trusted friend can help you with chores around the home. There are always people who are willing to help if you just ask.

304.   If you suffer from arthritis, you should monitor your weight. When you are overweight, more pressure is placed on your joints, increasing your discomfort. A healthier diet will not only reduce your weight but also make you feel better in general. Come up with a plan and have goals. Doing this will help you lose weight.

305.   Talk to your doctor before stopping or starting a medication. Changing medications can cause adverse effects, such as rebounding or a lack of tolerance.

306.   Keep in touch with your doctor about different options for treating your arthritis symptoms. There are almost always new options coming on the scene for treating arthritis. From new drugs to new physical therapies, stay on top

of these advances by making sure your doctor knows that you are interested in learning more and trying new options.

307.   Try to avoid taking pain killers for arthritis related pain. Prescriptions pain pills are often addictive and are used to temporarily treat your pain. Only use pain medications as prescribed, and under the supervision of your doctor.

308.   It is very important that you drink a lot of water and stay away from sugary drinks if you suffer from chronic arthritis. Water helps to improve muscle and joint strength, while sugary drinks like soda make you gain weight, which causes more pressure to be put on your joints.

309.   It may seem odd, but developing your abdominal muscles can prevent and reduce joint pain. Stronger abdominal muscles can improve your posture, which in turn can improve your joint health. When you work out, don't overdo it.

310.   Have a positive attitude. Negativity causes stress and depression, both of which can be very harmful to someone suffering from arthritis. Remove negative influences from your life, and learn to see the positive side of anything that

happens. Doing so will keep you going for much longer than if you let sadness overcome.

311.   Get educated about your unique condition. There are over a hundred different types of arthritis, and learning about yours will only help you be able to manage it more effectively. Get a diagnosis from a doctor, and then do your own research to find out what to expect and how to deal with it.

312.   Many people with arthritis become depressed because of their condition. It can alter many different aspects of their lives. Consider going to counseling to help you feel better. Counseling can help you identify problems in a way that will help you to think and act differently so that you can feel good about yourself.

313.   Do as much reading and researching as you can to learn about all the new innovations in arthritis therapy, both in the mainstream world of medicine and in a vast variety of alternative therapies. By knowing what's available to you, you will be able to create the most effective and creative therapy plan to address your arthritis pain needs.

314.   Be sure to keep yourself in the best physical condition possible. Even though, there is not currently a cure for arthritis, that does not mean there will never be. By maintaining your health and keeping fit, you are keeping yourself ready for that possibility. If-and-when a cure is found, you will be ready to try it successfully!

315.   It is important to get plenty of sleep. If you have problems doing this at night, then consider taking a nap during the day. If necessary, if you need a nap to get sufficient rest in the day, then schedule a nap routinely so you are sure to work it in.

316.   It is very important to keep good posture. Regardless of the things you put in your body or the amount of exercise you do, what really matters most when it comes to arthritis pain is your posture. When sitting, your back should be straight and your feel should be placed approximately one foot apart from each other. Doing this will ensure that you have correct posture, and you will easily minimize most of your joint stress along with the pain.

317.   You need to exercise when you have arthritis, though try to break your workouts into small segments. It might take you longer than

most people to exercise, but the benefits of exercise for your arthritis symptoms is proven with research. Complete 10 minutes of exercise at least three times a day to get maximum results.

318.   If you are hurting try alternating heat and cold. You can use hot and cold packs for instance. Once the hot packs stops having any effect on your arthritis, apply the cold one on the same spot. Repeat this operation until the pain is completely gone or at least attenuated.

319.   Omega 3s can help reduce the risks of arthritis. Omega 3s can be found in fish and oils. Make sure you include them in your diet, or take a supplement if you need to. This should prevent your arthritis from spreading and perhaps even reduce the pain you currently have.

320.   Most exercise programs for people who suffer from the pain and stiffness of arthritis include range-of-motion exercises. Range-of-motion is the normal amount of distance that your joints can move in a certain direction. These types of exercises help to keep your joints flexible. Some physicians also recommend Tai Chi as an alternative to improve flexibility and increase muscle strength.

321.	Give a vegetarian diet a try. Research has shown that individuals with arthritis who participate in this lifestyle often have less pain, less stiffness, and better grip strength than other people. If you are not ready to make this type of change, just try to eat more green foods. These foods can protect you from tissue damage.

322.	Take a warm bath or shower to relieve arthritis pain. The heat from the water should reduce stiffness in your joints and relax your tense muscles. Take as much time you need with the hot water and make sure that the room you're in has enough heat in it to stop your muscles from getting tighter after exiting the water

323.	If you are suffering from rheumatoid arthritis, make sure you're getting enough omega-3 in your diet. If you're not, consider taking a supplement like fish oil to help get those levels up. Studies have shown that omega-3 has many anti-inflammatory benefits for those who suffer from rheumatoid arthritis.

324.	Make sure you don't smoke. Smoking has been shown to increase your risk of developing rheumatoid arthritis. Not only that, but if you do develop it, smoking has been shown to worsen the joint damage. Patients who smoke most often have much more severe symptoms than those patients who don't smoke.

325.   Stay away from heating pads if your arthritis is flaring up. All they are going to do is make your symptoms worse. Instead, apply a cold compress to the area where your arthritis is located. You could even wrap a package of frozen peas or another frozen vegetable in a towel and apply to the area.

326.   Learn all you can about arthritis to stay proactive about managing your disease. There are a host of useful resources covering everything from nutrition to pain management for arthritis sufferers. If you take the time to educate yourself about arthritis, there is a good chance you will find all kinds of great things to help yourself out.

327.   Get in the water. Water aerobics is a great low impact exercise for arthritis sufferers, because not only does it put minimal strain on joints, it also provides resistance for strengthening. If you are uncomfortable with doing these in large groups, learn a few moves and take to the pool. You will quickly become more comfortable.

328.   Many people tend to have bad posture and do all sorts of things that wreak havoc on their bodies. When you have arthritis, it is even more important to pay close attention to things like this. You need to make sure you maintain good posture and the correct positioning of your body.

329.   Sometimes, the treatments that your doctor offers for arthritis can be assisted and enhanced with alternative treatments such as hydrotherapy, yoga, hot and cold therapy or some herbal or dietary supplements. Be sure to ask your doctor about alternative treatments that will help you make the most of your arthritis care.

330.   By staying fit and active, you will help your arthritis to remain at bay. If weightlifting isn't an option, then try resistance exercises, like water aerobics. The water will give you support and will massage your muscles as you are doing the exercises. Water therapy is a surefire way to help manage arthritis.

331.   Be sure to get regular exercise as part of your arthritis therapy. Avoid exercise that stresses your joints, such as aerobics, running, and possibly, bicycling. Instead, try water aerobics, swimming, and possibly, yoga. These forms of

exercise minimize pressure on the joints and maximize flexibility. Remember not to overdo exercise. Give your body ample time to rest and recover.

332.   Ask a dietician about what foods have anti-inflammatory properties. He or she will suggest a diet full of Omega three and six fatty acids. This will help to keep your weight at an optimum level. Find out as much as possible about foods that are helpful in treating and alleviating the symptoms and pain of arthritis.

333.   Youngsters who have juvenile rheumatoid arthritis must be encouraged to visit a physical therapist on a regular basis to establish and maintain an exercise program. Frequent follow-ups will keep this program properly adjusted to the child's current abilities. A good physical therapy program should include: range-of-motion, strength training and endurance training.

334.   Nutrition is necessary for a healthy life, and this is especially true for arthritis sufferers. Diets that put their emphasis on fresh fruits and vegetables, legumes and essential oils like olive oil will have an amazing impact on how the body functions naturally, as well as increasing its vitality. You can ditch those arthritic symptoms

by staying fit and healthy. A good, balanced diet will give you a boost of energy, and you will subsequently have the energy to stay fit and fight your arthritis.

335.   Gentle stretching exercises or yoga are an excellent way for arthritis sufferers to get up and move without injuring themselves. Keeping your body limber can help you avoid injuries that are common in people with joint problems, and it will also increase your energy levels and help your body stay healthy.

336.   Meditation can be highly effective in coping with arthritis. The brain is an often overlooked tool in dealing with disease or debilitating conditions. Through meditation you can condition your mind to work for you. You can achieve relaxed states in which you create mantras that program your thinking in regards to how you deal with pain and stress.

337.   Regular exercise can help you manage the pain which is associated with arthritis. Your doctor can recommend an exercise program for you. Some physicians elect to send their arthritis patients to a physical therapist or an occupational therapist to have them design an exercise program for them to follow.

338.   Stop and go! Arthritis can be tough! You want to get enough rest to feel comfortable and pain-free, but not so much that your joints stiffen up and become painful. Resting can ease your pain and give you a break from the stress. Find a happy balance between the amount of exercise you need and the amount of rest you need every day.

339.   Pay close attention to the strength of your muscles around the knees and the quadriceps. Spend time with a trainer to learn the safest ways for you to help work on these important muscle groups. Your hip and thigh are also a great area to work on as well.